PERFECT BODY FORMULA

A guide to maintaining the perfect body weight through dieting

LEONARD S. GRANT

TABLE OF CONTENT

INTRODUCTION

An overall expansion in overweight and heftiness, weight-the-board through the way of life changes has turned into a significant general medical problem. Youths and youthful grown-ups contain a weak gathering. The progress into adulthood addresses a phase in life while laying out a great way of life propensities for what's to come is significant. The point of this study was to investigate inspiration and impediments for weight decrease, weight upkeep, and sound way of life decisions in young ladies. Before you start on a tight eating routine and wellness plan, there are a couple of inquiries that you ought to pose.

Do I Need To Lose Weight?

This might appear to be senseless or self-evident, however, your PCP can inform you as to whether you really need to get more fit. You may not really be overweight. Getting in shape when it's superfluous can prompt a large group of clinical issues. Your weight the board doctor can assist you with staying away from that.

The amount of Weight I Need To Lose?

When you realize that you really want to shed pounds, your PCP can assist you with deciding the amount you really want to lose. This assists you with laying out an objective, however, it keeps you more secure. A specialist can see how much weight you really need to lose and ensure that you don't go overboard.

Is My Current Weight Affecting My Health?

Assuming that you're overweight or fat, your weight could be causing other clinical issues. A portion of these issues can improve on the off chance that you get in shape, which can give you an objective to pursue.

What Should I Eat and How Much Of It Should I Eat?

The vast majority have close to zero insight into good dieting, however, your primary care physician realizes definitely more than you do. They can suggest explicit food varieties in light of your set of experiences, what drugs you're taking, and what other medical problems you're at present managing. A doctor can likewise tell you a sound number of calories to consume.

Will My Medications Affect My Weight Loss Plan?

Talking about medicine, a few doctor-prescribed medications can really unfavorably affect your weight reduction endeavors. Meds going from antidepressants to beta blockers might possibly cause weight gain and obstruct your endeavors.

Is Surgery An Option?

Contingent upon your wellness level, a careful weight reduction method could be a choice. Your primary care physician can make sense of why it would work for you and let you in on the likely dangers. The person in question can likewise update you on what a weight reduction medical procedure means for your life. Careful choices generally mean severe dietary norms. On the off chance that you don't imagine that you can adhere to them, then, at that point, this probably won't be the ideal decision for you.

The amount of Exercise Is Healthy For Me?

If you're attempting to shed pounds, exercise can help. Various sorts of activity request more energy and actual capacity be that as it may, and your PCP can assist you with sorting out what sort of activity routine is sound and the amount of it you can deal with.

KEEPING UP WITH A HEALTHY DIET

A solid eating routine assists with safeguarding against unhealthiness in the entirety of its structures, as well as noncommunicable illnesses, including; diabetes, coronary illness, stroke, and disease.

Unfortunate eating regimens and the absence of actual work are driving worldwide dangers to well-being.

Solid dietary practices start right off the bat throughout everyday life - breastfeeding encourages sound development and works on the mental turn of events, and may have longer-term medical advantages like diminishing the gamble of becoming overweight or fat and creating NCDs further down the road.

Energy consumption (calories) ought to be offset with energy use. To keep away from undesirable weight gain, all-out fat shouldn't surpass 30% of complete energy admission.

Admission of immersed fats ought to be under 10% of complete energy admission, and admission of trans-fats under 1% of all out energy admission, with a change in fat utilization away from soaked fats and trans-fats

to unsaturated fats, and towards the objective of disposing of mechanically created trans-fats.
Restricting admission of free sugars to under 10% of complete energy consumption is important for a solid eating routine. A further decrease to under 5% of complete energy admission is proposed for extra medical advantages.
Keeping salt admission to under 5 g each day (comparable to sodium admission of under 2 g each day) assists with forestalling hypertension, and decreases the gamble of coronary illness and stroke in the grown-up populace.
WHO the Member States have consented to decrease the worldwide populace's admission of salt by 30% by 2025; they have additionally consented to end the ascent in diabetes and corpulence in grown-ups and young people as well as in youth overweight by 2025.
Outline
Nonetheless, the expanded creation of handled food varieties, fast urbanization, and changing ways of life have prompted a change in dietary examples. Individuals are currently devouring more food varieties high in energy, fats, free sugars, and salt/sodium, and many individuals don't eat enough natural products, vegetables, and

other dietary fibers like entire grains.
The specific make-up of an enhanced, adjusted and sound eating routine will change contingent upon individual qualities (for example age, orientation, way of life, and level of actual work), social setting, locally accessible food varieties, and dietary traditions. Be that as it may, the essential standards of what is a solid eating routine continue as before.

For grown-ups

A sound eating routine incorporates the accompanying:
Natural products, vegetables, vegetables (for example lentils and beans), nuts, and entire grains (for example natural maize, millet, oats, wheat, and earthy colored rice).
No less than 400 g (for example five parts) of foods grown from the ground each day, barring potatoes, yams, cassava, and other boring roots.
Under 10% of complete energy consumption from free sugars, which is identical to 50 g (or around 12 level teaspoons) for an individual of solid body weight consuming around 2000 calories

each day, yet preferably is under 5% of all out energy admission for extra medical advantages. Free sugars are sugars added to food varieties or beverages by the maker, cook, or purchaser, as well as sugars normally present in honey, syrups, natural product squeezes, and natural product juice condensed.

Under 30% of absolute energy consumption is from fats. Unsaturated fats (tracked down in fish, avocado, and nuts, and in sunflower, soybean, canola, and olive oils) are desirable over soaked fats (found in greasy meat, margarine, palm and coconut oil, cream, cheddar, ghee, and fat) and trans-fats, all things considered, including both mechanically created trans-fats (tracked down in heated and broiled food varieties, and pre-bundled bites and food varieties, like frozen pizza, pies, treats, bread rolls, wafers, and cooking oils and spreads) and ruminant trans-fats (tracked down in meat and dairy food sources from ruminant creatures, like cows, sheep, goats, and camels). It is recommended that the admission of immersed fats be diminished to under 10% of all out energy consumption and trans-fats to under 1% of absolute energy consumption. Specifically, economically delivered trans-fats

are not a piece of a solid eating routine and ought to stay away from.
Under g of salt (identical to around one teaspoon) each day.. Salt ought to be iodized.

For Babies and small kids

In the initial 2 years of a kid's life, ideal sustenance cultivates sound development and works on the mental turn of events. It additionally lessens the gamble of becoming overweight or hefty and creating NCDs further down the road.
Exhortation on a solid eating regimen for babies and kids is like that for grown-ups, however, the accompanying components are additionally significant:
Newborn children ought to be breastfed solely during the initial half year of life. Newborn children ought to be breastfed persistently until 2 years old and then some. From a half-year-old enough, bosom milk ought to be supplemented with various sufficient, protected, and supplement thick food sources. Salt and sugars ought not to be added to corresponding food sources.

Pragmatic exhortation on keeping a sound eating regimen. Eating no less than 400 g, or five segments, of products of the soil each day, decreases the gamble of NCDs and assists with guaranteeing a sufficient everyday admission of dietary fiber.

Products of the soil admission can be improved by:

continuously remembering vegetables for dinners;

eating new products of the soil vegetables as bites;

eating new products of the soil that are in season; and

eating an assortment of leafy foods.

Fats

Diminishing how much all-out fat admission to under 30% of complete energy consumption assists with forestalling undesirable weight gain in the grown-up populace.. Likewise, the gamble of creating NCDs is brought down by:

Diminishing immersed fats to under 10% of absolute energy admission;

decreasing trans-fats to under 1% of all out energy admission; and

supplanting both immersed fats and trans-fats with unsaturated fats - specifically, with polyunsaturated fats.

Fat admission, particularly immersed fat and economically

created trans-fat admission, can be diminished by:

Steaming or bubbling as opposed to searing while cooking;

Supplanting margarine, grease, and ghee with oils wealthy in polyunsaturated fats, like soybean, canola (rapeseed), corn, safflower, and sunflower oils;

eating decreased fat dairy food sources and lean meats, or cutting back apparent excess from meat; and

restricting the utilization of heated and broiled food varieties, and pre-bundled bites and food sources (for example doughnuts, cakes, pies, treats, rolls, and wafers) that contain economically created trans-fats.

Salt, sodium, and potassium

The vast majority consume a lot of sodium through salt (relating to consuming a normal of 9-12 g of salt each day) and insufficient potassium. High sodium consumption and lacking potassium admission add to hypertension, which thusly builds the gamble of coronary illness and stroke.

Decreasing salt admission to the suggested degree of under 5 g each day could forestall 1.7 million passings every year. Individuals are frequently uninformed about how much salt they consume. In numerous nations, most salt comes from handled food varieties (for example prepared feasts; handled meats like bacon, ham, and salami; cheddar; and pungent tidbits) or from food varieties devoured regularly in enormous sums (for example bread). Salt is additionally added to food varieties during cooking (for example bouillon, stock 3D shapes, soy sauce, and fish sauce) or at the place of utilization (for example table salt).

Salt admission can be decreased by:

Restricting how much salt and high-sodium sauces (for example soy sauce, fish sauce, and bouillon) while cooking and planning food varieties;

not having salt or high-sodium sauces on the table;

restricting the utilization of pungent tidbits; and

picking items with lower sodium content.

Some food makers are reformulating recipes to lessen the sodium content of their items, and individuals ought to be urged to check nourishment names to perceive how much sodium is in an item before buying or devouring it. Potassium can alleviate the adverse consequences of raised sodium utilization on the circulatory strain. Admission of potassium can be expanded by consuming new foods grown from the ground.

Sugar

In the two grown-ups and youngsters, the admission of free sugars ought to be diminished to under 10% of all our energy consumption. A decrease to under 5% of all out energy admission would give extra medical advantages. Consuming free sugars expands the gamble of dental caries (tooth rot). The overabundance of calories from food varieties and savors with high free sugars additionally add to undesirable weight gain, which can prompt overweight and stoutness. Late proof likewise shows that free sugars impact circulatory strain and serum lipids, and recommends that a decrease in free sugars consumption diminishes risk factors for cardiovascular illnesses.

Sugars admission can be decreased by:

restricting the utilization of food sources and beverages containing high measures of sugars, for example, sweet bites, confections, and sugar-improved drinks (for example a wide range of refreshments containing free sugars - these incorporate carbonated or non-carbonated soda pops, natural products or vegetable squeezes and beverages, fluid and powder concentrates, seasoned water, energy and sports drinks, ready-to-drink tea, ready-to-drink espresso, and enhanced milk drinks); and

eating new leafy foods and vegetables as snacks rather than sweet bites.

Diet develops after some time, being impacted by numerous social and financial variables that collaborate in a complicated way to shape individual dietary examples. These variables incorporate pay, food costs (which will influence the accessibility and moderation of good food sources), individual inclinations and convictions, social customs, and topographical and natural perspectives (counting environmental change). Consequently, advancing a quality food climate - including food frameworks that advance an enhanced, adjusted, and solid eating routine - requires the inclusion of numerous areas and partners, including government, general society, and confidential areas. States play a focal part in establishing a good food climate that empowers individuals to embrace and keep up with sound dietary practices. Viable activities by strategy creators to establish a quality food climate incorporate the accompanying:

Making lucidness in public strategies and growth strategies - including exchange, food, and farming arrangements - to advance a sound eating routine and safeguard general wellbeing through:

expanding impetuses for makers and retailers to develop, use and sell new leafy foods;

decreasing motivations for the food business to proceed or build the creation of handled food varieties containing elevated degrees of immersed fats, trans-fats, free sugars, and salt/sodium;

empowering reformulation of food items to lessen the items in immersed fats, trans-fats, free sugars, and salt/sodium, fully intent on disposing of economically created trans-fats;

executing the WHO suggestions on the promoting of food varieties and non-cocktails to youngsters;

laying out guidelines to cultivate solid dietary practices through guaranteeing the accessibility of sound, nutritious, protected, and reasonable food varieties in pre-schools, schools, other public foundations, and the work environment;

investigating administrative and deliberate instruments,and financial impetuses or disincentives to advance a solid eating routine; and empowering transnational, public, and nearby food administrations and cooking outlets to work on the wholesome nature of their food varieties - guaranteeing the accessibility and reasonableness of solid decisions - and survey segment sizes and valuing.

Empowering customer interest in good food sources and feasts through:

Creating school strategies and projects that urge kids to embrace and keep a sound eating regimen;

teaching kids, teenagers, and grown-ups about nourishment and solid dietary practices;

empowering culinary abilities, remembering for kids through schools;

supporting retail location data, including through nourishment naming that guarantees precise, normalized, and fathomable data on supplement contents in food varieties (following the Codex Alimentarius Commission rules), with the expansion of front-of-pack marking to work with customer understanding; and

giving sustenance and dietary guidance at essential medical services offices.

Advancing fitting baby and small kid taking care of practices through:

executing the International Code of Marketing of Breast-milk

Substitutes and ensuing pertinent World Health Assembly goals;
executing arrangements and practices to advance insurance of working moms; and
advancing, securing, and supporting breastfeeding in well-being administrations and the local area, including through the Baby-accommodating Hospital Initiative.

PERFECT WEIGHT

A solid weight is a number that is related to generally safe weight-related infections and medical problems. Albeit solid weight rules have been created at populace levels, every individual's sound weight territory will change and rely upon elements, for example, age, sex, hereditary qualities, body outline, existing clinical history, way of life propensities, and weight as a youthful grown-up. Weight is only one of the numerous determinants of well-being. Weight list (BMI), which estimates weight normalized for level, is much of the time utilized as a proportion of wellbeing risk. Even though it doesn't gauge muscle-to-fat ratio or body structure straightforwardly, research has shown BMI to connect intimately with different strategies that straightforwardly measure muscle-to-fat ratio.

How valuable are the MET Life Height-Weigh Tables?

There are many purposes behind weight gain including specific prescriptions (corticosteroids, antidepressants, beta-blockers, antipsychotics, insulin), pregnancy, constant pressure, persistently unfortunate rest, an inordinate calorie admission, and absence of sufficient activity.
It is useful to keep a consistent load however much as could be expected and control inordinate weight gain after some time, which is unequivocally connected with well-being gambles.

Keep up with, Don't Gain

Keeping a solid weight can bring down the gamble of coronary illness, stroke, diabetes, hypertension, and a wide range of tumors. Your weight, abdomen size, and how much weight acquired since your mid-20s can have well-being suggestions around the waist. Qualities don't need to become predetermination, in any case, and studies recommend that eating a sound eating routine, remaining dynamic, and staying away from undesirable propensities like drinking soft drinks can forestall the hereditary inclination to gamble for heftiness. Peruse more about hereditary gamble for corpulence on the Obesity Prevention Source.

Actual idleness

The practice has a large group of medical advantages, including lessening the possibilities of creating coronary illness, a few kinds of malignant growth, and other constant infections. Actual work is a critical component of weight control and well-being.
Stress. Persistent pressure can prompt undesirable dietary patterns, for example, raised cortisol levels causing desires for "solace" food sources of exceptionally handled tidbits or desserts, having the lower inspiration to plan adjusted feasts or in any event, neglecting to eat, and upsetting rest that can prompt higher admissions of

caffeine or fatty sweet snacks to help energy.

Deficient rest. The research proposes that there's a connection between how much individuals rest and the amount they gauge. As a general rule, youngsters and grown-ups who get too little rest will quite often weigh more than the individuals who get sufficient rest.

the plate of cheddar puff snacks close to a TV screen to connote publicizing unhealthy food

The impact of our surroundings

However significant as individual decisions seem to be concerning wellbeing, nobody individual acts in a vacuum. The physical and social climate where individuals reside assumes a gigantic part in the food and action decisions they make. Sadly, in the U.S. also, progressively all over the planet, our surroundings are not streamlined for sound living. From the determined promotion and accessibility of unfortunate food sources and sweet beverages to time and well-being imperatives for remaining dynamic, people are confronted with different difficulties. Heftiness and its causes have, in numerous ways, become woven into the texture of our general public. To effectively unravel them will adopt a diverse strategy that not just gives individuals the ability to go with better decisions yet in addition sets set up a strategy and foundation that help those decisions.

Advantages of Even Modest Weight Loss

Assuming you have acquired more than 25 pounds in adulthood, losing that weight might appear to be overwhelming. What's more, when the additional weight doesn't feel quite a bit better, you might be enticed to begin an exceptional weight-reduction plan. In any case, fortunately even an unassuming weight reduction of 5% of your ongoing body weight is probably going to deliver a few medical advantages, remembering upgrades for your pulse, blood cholesterol, blood sugars, actual portability, and personal satisfaction.

KEEPING UP WITH THE PERFECT WEIGHT

Keep it without rushing. Individuals who get in shape bit by bit and consistently (around 1 to 2 pounds each week) are more fruitful at keeping weight off. This permits the body to acclimate to the change and can bring down the gamble of areas of strength for creating sensations of hardship that frequently go with more fast weight reduction.

Incorporate self-administration and observation. This incorporates laying out objectives, for example, with the SMART abbreviation, which represents Specific, Measurable, Achievable, Relevant, and Time-Bound. Begin by making 2-3 momentary SMART objectives. Self-observing, for example, with day-to-day or week-by-week food journaling or utilizing conduct applications can give knowledge and responsibility to eating ways of behaving. This classification likewise incorporates critical thinking, for example, having an arrangement for "backslides" if weight is recovered because of upsetting life-altering events, occasions, or occupation requests.

Make an emotionally supportive network. The research proposes that having successive contact with others for help (e.g., believed relative or companion, doctor, wellbeing mentor, enlisted dietitian, or an individual companion or colleague on a comparative solid weight venture) can be important in giving consolation and responsibility.

Foster smart dieting designs. Albeit a few scientists have scrutinized the value of energy balance (calories eaten versus calories consumed), current proof shows that calorie decrease stays the best methodology for weight control. There are numerous dietary techniques (e.g., high-carb low-fat versus low-carb high-fat versus discontinuous fasting versus a Mediterranean eating routine), however, research has not predictably shown more prominent weight reduction with one arrangement over one more in the long haul. The Healthy Eating Plate model that gives adjusted nourishment and part control is a decent spot to begin.

Practice care. Do you eat excessively quick or while diverted sitting in front of the TV or looking at your telephone? Do you stretch eat or nibble in any event, when not ravenous? Careful eating tends to these ways of behaving that are related to weight gain. Expanding mindfulness and enthusiasm for food can give more prominent fulfillment, genuinely and intellectually, that might assist with decreasing gorging.

Remain dynamic. Practice is one part of keeping a sound weight and forestalling weight gain, however, it likewise assumes a critical part in prosperity and psychological well-being. The National Weight Control Registry, which follows individuals who have lost and kept a 30-pound misfortune for no less than one year, shows that members incorporate around one hour of moderate-energetic work-out day to day like lively strolling. Anyway, there is variety among members, with a few requiring more activity and some less to keep the load off. How much is required will rely upon one's qualities and way of life factors? Performing various sorts of activities can grow the scope of advantages considerably further.

Focus on taking care of oneself. In a surged society with endless requests, dealing with our bodies can rapidly tumble to the lower part of our need list. Committing time to really focus on one's close-to-home, physical, and otherworldly necessities can advance a solid weight. Large numbers of the elements recorded above are instances of taking care of oneself; others could be finding another side interest, rehearsing day-to-day contemplation, or permitting time to simply sit idle. Taking care of oneself might assist with further developing a mindset and a feeling of prosperity, and increment inspiration and energy levels. It likewise develops self-empathy and versatility, as one figures out how to acknowledge their error and continue on.

Cell phones or versatile wellbeing applications are self-checking effectively open apparatuses individuals can use to follow their weight and dietary admission. Self-observing is firmly connected with self-viability, characterized as an individual believing in their capacity to work on one's wellbeing by evolving ways of behaving. Individuals can utilize these applications to survey their wholesome admission by logging explicit food sources and eating designs. Applications might give a food information base from which to look, a photograph capability to take pictures of feasts, and a filtering device to find food items utilizing standardized tags, or food symbols. Other applications screen eating ways of behaving, for example, stress-related or profound eating, eating rapidly or on the run, and gorging. A significant advantage of these devices is expanded familiarity with sorts of food varieties eaten and eating ways of behaving that could be adding to weight gain or changes in metabolic boundaries like high blood glucose or cholesterol.

The quantity of wellbeing-related applications focusing on conduct change has blasted, with more than 325,000 applications economically accessible in 2017. Wellbeing applications are in many cases minimal expense or free and can be successful at-home observing devices that supplement conventional considerations like face-to-face visits to a specialist or dietitian. For instance, on the off chance that a medical services supplier encourages a patient to get thinner to further develop a persistent ailment, a nourishing application can give the following, responsibility, and connection that draws in the patient until the following medical care supplier visit.

This might be particularly helpful for specific gatherings; one investigation discovered that countrymen were bound to effectively utilize well-being applications for weight reduction/sustenance programs than to take part in up close and personal projects, because of social standards of confidence. Meta-examinations show that individuals who use applications can encounter more prominent weight reduction, diminished abdomen circuit, and lower calorie admission contrasted and controls, for the time being. Different examinations have shown benefits in further developing sustenance ways of behaving, pulse, and blood cholesterol. however, there are constraints to these meta-investigations that made correlations troublesome: the investigations utilized different business applications with shifting capabilities, and members utilized the applications at different levels (e.g., day to day versus week after week). Likewise, the greater part of the examinations was of brief term at under a half year. For the most part, the more frequently the application was utilized, the more prominent adherence there was to healthful objectives and accomplishing weight reduction. Tragically a significant number of the examinations proposed that application utilization commonly declined after some time. In any case, well-being applications merit a pursue anybody beginning a solid way of life plan and for the people who probably won't have simple admittance to other emotionally supportive networks.

Everybody knows the famous weight reduction mantra: Move more and eat less. Furthermore, even though they're recorded together, these two recommendations needn't bother with to be dealt with similarly. It is feasible to get thinner without a workout. Allow us to make sense of it.

Priorities straight: we are not rejecting that moderate-power practice is great for keeping up with and working on your wellbeing; in any case, many examinations have uncovered proof that practice alone may not be the most ideal way to get more fit.

Many weight reduction methodologies recommend that the more you figure out, the more calories you'll consume, and the more you'll shed pounds. However, a new report distributed in Current Biology found that this may not be valid. The specialists found that once you begin working out consistently, your body might wind up adjusting to this new degree of action. Subsequently, your body might wind up bringing down the all-out number of calories it needs.

"There is lots of proof that exercise is significant for keeping our bodies and brains solid, and this work never really changes that message," one of the review's creators, Professor Herman Pontzer of City University of New York, told The

Guardian. "What our work adds is that we likewise need to zero in on diet, especially with regards to dealing with our weight and forestalling or turning around unfortunate weight gain."

Significantly more examination shows exercise can subvert weight reduction by making you hungrier and it can misdirect you into believing it's alright to enjoy low-quality foods either as a prize for practicing or because you've made a calorie shortfall. One Obesity Reviews investigation even discovered that individuals will generally misjudge the number of calories they that copy when they exercise. Subsequently, members ordinarily overcompensated for their exercises by eating a bigger number of calories than they consumed.

Even though exercise can unquestionably assist with building fat-consuming muscle, it may not shrivel your waistline however much changing your eating regimen will.

So since it has become so undeniably obvious that "eating less" ought to take need in your weight reduction venture, where to begin? Since it's not exactly simple or easy, we've revealed some thinning privileged insights that can assist you with dropping pounds through diet trades as well as way of life and dietary pattern changes. (Furthermore, indeed, de-focusing on an air pocket shower is one of them.) Read on to figure out how to get thinner quickly without working out, and for more on the most proficient method to practice good eating habits, you won't have any desire to miss these 21 Best Healthy Cooking Hacks of All Time.

PERFECT WEIGHT FORMULA

Need to eat less? Your most memorable line of protection is getting a decent night's rest. At the point when you don't get sufficient quality closed eyes, your body expands levels of the craving chemical ghrelin and diminishes the satiety chemical leptin — bringing about unignorable food cravings. Also, concentrates on the show that your restless self needs more unfortunate, unhealthy, and high-fat food sources, and that implies you'll eat more food, yet you'll eat more garbage. For additional ways of getting more fit around evening time, read up — then ditch — these evening propensities that cause weight gain.

Take Your Coffee Black

More than 50% of Americans drink espresso consistently, and a considerable lot of them use calorie-loaded added substances like sugar, enhanced syrups, or cream in their refreshment. Thus, as opposed to being a zero or five-calorie drink, the typical carbohydrate content of a cuppa joe skyrockets 1,280 percent, to 69 calories, as per a new report distributed in the diary Public Health. Not exclusively will taking your espresso dark save you almost 500 calories per week, however, since more than 60% of those calories come from sugar, you'll likewise be bringing down your gamble of insulin opposition, diabetes, and other metabolic issues. Leaving the sugar parcels on the rack is one of our simple methods for cutting calories.

Convey a Water Bottle Everywhere

Did you have at least some idea that 60% of the time we improperly answer thirst by eating as opposed to drinking? So says a concentrate in the diary Physiology and Behavior. Specialists accept the misstep comes from the way that a similar piece of our mind controls yearning and thirst, and once in a while it stirs up the signs. Not exclusively will keeping a water bottle around assist you with answering thirst accurately, yet chugging water can assist you with feeling full, keep your digestion murmuring, and even assist you to debloat!

Change From Canola Oil to Extra-Virgin Olive Oil

Vegetable oils like canola and soybean oil are high in fiery omega-6 unsaturated fats, which can toss your body into a condition of constant irritation, causing weight gain and skin issues. All things considered, snatch a jug of additional virgin olive oil, whose polyphenols have been known to assist with bringing down circulatory strain and whose oleic corrosive has been found to assist with decreasing craving and advancing weight reduction.

Choose 2% pouring milk

Dairy fat, that is. You might be shocked to hear it, yet without fat food doesn't guarantee to mean a sans-fat body; According to a European Journal of Nutrition study, members who ate full-fat dairy would in general weigh less and put on less weight over the long haul than the people who decided on non-fat items. Specialists make sense that non-fat food sources can be less fulfilling generally speaking thanks to the low-fat substance (since fats are processed gradually and can keep you full longer) and because many sans-fat food things are made with midsection broadening fake fixings.

Stash a Snack in Your Bag

Try not to push through that mid-evening protest. Believe us. Investigations have discovered that the people who eat delayed snacks, and the people who go the most in the middle between dinners wind up consuming more calories during those feasts contrasted with the individuals who eat on a more regular basis. The thinking is basic: when you're ravenous — and running on void — your body changes to starvation mode and builds the creation of your appetite chemicals, which then makes you overcompensate at your next feast. To hold yourself back from gorging, consistently convey a nibble with you.

Give Healthy Foods Prime Shelf Space

The unhealthy food battle is genuine — we know. Also, a determination isn't to be faulted. A University of Sydney investigation discovered that eating low-quality food can turn into a propensity and one that is sustained basically by venturing into a room (like your kitchen) or encountering a food prompt (like a cheap food business). Ending these terrible dietary patterns will take time and persistence, yet there's a basic fix: Prioritize quality food varieties before unhealthy food in your storage room. For that, while you're wanting a treat you need to shove aside the almonds and quinoa to get to it. It'll act as a little wake-up call to keep up your better-body objectives.

Keep Chopped Veggies On Hand hacked veggies

Top off on veggies and you'll be less inclined to finish up your pants. Research distributed in the diary PLOS Medicine connected more noteworthy utilization of high-fiber vegetables to more prominent weight reduction results when contrasted and eating less low in high-fiber food sources. In addition to the fact that these veggies super-satisfying are, they're additionally brimming with mitigating cancer prevention agents and will uproot snacks like supplements lacking potato chips and pretzels.

Make At Least One of Your Meals Meatless

You don't need to go full-scale veggie lover to receive the rewards of a without-meat diet. Simply pursue one lunch or supper seven days to get thinner without working out. In doing as such, you'll be consuming more plant-based protein, which a

University of Copenhagen concentrates on and observed to be much more fulfilling than pork and veal-based dinners, and cause individuals to feel all the more full. It improves: The scientists likewise found that members who ate a vegan high-protein dinner consumed 12% fewer calories in their next feast contrasted with the people who ate meat!

Keep a Stocked Freezer

full cooler

You have two choices when you return home late from work starving and see a vacant refrigerator — one, request gut swelling, unhealthy, oily takeout, or two, prepare a fast veggie-pressed pan sear with the frozen veggies you generally keep in your cooler. If you keep sound fixings close by (like frozen organic products, veggies, and pre-partitioned protein), you will not need to fall back on unfortunate conveyance dinners. For tips on what you ought to stock in your storeroom, don't miss these weight reduction fixings to continuously have available.

Kick the Can

One of the least complex ways of slicing calories is to restrict items that have added sugar. These basic carbs are drained of supplements and can make you ceaselessly eager (and that implies you're probably going to the gorge). The best strategy is to focus on refreshments: sweet espressos, teas, and pop. These fluid calories are on a whole other level: An American Journal of Clinical Nutrition found that energy got from drinking liquids has been demonstrated to be less fulfilling than calories from strong food varieties, which makes us drink more (and a more prominent number of calories) before we feel.

fulfilled. Just to perceive how ineffectively your number one stacks up among the pack, look at our restrictive report: well-known soft drinks positioned by nourishment.

Earthy colored Bag It

Setting up your lunch implies you put the calorie-cutting power in your own hands — not in that frame of mind of the restaurateurs who have no stake in your weight reduction venture. Set up any of these solid snacks under 400 calories, and you'll save 600 calories a dinner contrasted with on the off chance that you ate at a standard semi-formal eatery, whose late morning feast has an average of over 1,100 calories.

Free Yourself From Your Desk

A mid-day break ought to be only that — a break! Research

distributed in the American Journal of Clinical Nutrition found that youngsters who eat while occupied (like while watching T.V.) can consume 218 calories more at a time than they would somehow. Specialists make sense that keeping your psyche occupied while eating can keep specific satiety signals from educating your cerebrum that you've had your fill.

Make Your Meals Gram-Worthy

You will not simply get more likes on your Instagram photograph. Making your food look picture-wonderful can urge you to stack your plate up with additional brilliant, new veggies. Additionally, it might try and make your food taste better! A review distributed in the diary Health Psychology found that when members invested energy in setting up the food they make, they viewed it as fundamentally more fulfilling than the people who had the food arranged for them, regardless of whether the food was thought of as "solid."

Have you ever known about the fish diet? You see food and promptly eat it! To control your low-quality food utilization, begin by freeing your work area and kitchen counters of your dietary kryptonite. Keeping these indecencies noticeable will get you in a position for disappointment by setting off a characteristic named by Oxford specialists as "visual yearning:" a transformative quality that expands levels of craving chemicals when we see food. All things being equal, conceal your reserve in obscure compartments or toward the rear of your bureau.

Cheerful Without Happy Hours Every Day

See, we'll be quick to let you know we love wine — particularly red wine, which offers cell reinforcements and is viewed as moderately sound when polished off with some restraint (something like two glasses every day). Be that as it may, on the off chance that you're hoping to get more fit, one of our best tips is to put down the glass. Since liquor is genuinely caloric and gives moderately scarcely any nourishing advantages, drinking ought not to be an ordinary occasion. For instance, two pints of lager daily can add almost 2,000 calories to your week-after-week consumption — so removing it can assist you with shedding more than two pounds every month. For those couple of times that you in all actuality do decide to enjoy, however, do so carefully with the assistance of these ways to pick sound cocktails.

Take Half to Go

We approve of eating out once in a little while, however, regarding this exhortation: request that your server takes care of a portion of the dinner before it arrives at the table. A Journal of the Academy of Nutrition and Dietetics concentrate on found that the normal dinner at your neighborhood American, Chinese, or Italian eatery contains an incredible 1,500 calories, so following this tip can save you a cool 750 calories. Furthermore, you'll get a free lunch later!

Continuously Sub Fries for A Side Salad

We're singing, "bye, bye, miss American fries!" You could stay with your week-after-week burger request from your number one bar, simply sub out the spuds for a serving of mixed greens. Doing so can save more than 150 calories while topping you off with fiber-rich veggies that are perfect for working on stomach-related well-being.

Serve Yourself

Here is a straightforward tip to try not to eat unfortunate food varieties: serve yourself. As indicated by USC specialists, the straightforward demonstration of plating your grub, rather than having a server or companion dole out aid for you, can control an unfortunate guilty pleasure. So whenever you're commending a collaborator's birthday, serve (and cut!) your cut of the cake.

Have An Intimate Dinner

Here is an extraordinary reason for a night out!: another Cornell investigation discovered that men are at a one-of-a-kind gamble of gorging in friendly circumstances — regardless of whether there is not a motivation to do such. "Regardless of whether men aren't mulling over everything, eating more than a companion will, in general, be perceived as an exhibition of virility and strength," made sense of co-creator of the review, Kevin Kniffin, Ph.D. So rather than meeting up with an entire group for an evening out on the town, settle on a heartfelt supper for two or see your companions each, in turn, to hold yourself back from getting out of hand.

Attempt a New Recipe

Solace food varieties procure a spot in our souls since they taste great and bring serious areas of strength to our, recollections of growing up. Even though it's OK to enjoy one of these works of art once in a little while, you might need to eliminate the number of mother's recipes in your week-after-week roundup. As indicated by an investigation of 30 years of information by the London School of Economics, the conventional dinners your folks and grandparents used to make are essentially excessively caloric for our less-dynamic age. All things being equal, don't hesitate for even a moment to branch out of your usual range of familiarity and look at better recipes: begin with these 20 Healthy Sandwich Recipes!

Pass on "Diet" Foods

It can appear to be a straightforward fix while you're starting a new and improved eating routine, however, don't succumb to these showcasing ploys. "Diet" food varieties are typically stacked with counterfeit sugars like sucralose and aspartame. Albeit misleadingly improved refreshments contain fewer calories than sweet renditions, a survey of over 30 years of studies viewed there as no strong proof that sugar choices forestall weight gain. Albeit misleadingly improved refreshments contain fewer calories than sweet adaptations, specialists say they trigger sweet receptors in the cerebrum, which might cause individuals to hunger for food. Combined with the way that a great many people view diet drinks as better, it could prompt over-utilization, the specialists contend.

Cook Your Food

You realize that eatery dishes are high in calories, however, we're not simply discussing takeout. A review distributed in the diary BMJ Open found that most food Americans eat is "super handled," and that implies an item is made of a few handled fixings like flavors, colors, sugars, emulsifiers, and different added substances to camouflage its unfortunate characteristics. Models incorporate locally acquired things like bread, frozen dinners, pop, pizza, and breakfast cereals. Not in the least do super-handled food varieties need supplements that safeguard against medical problems, they make up 90% of our added sugar consumption, which makes a scope of medical problems from corpulence type II diabetes. Sub out a Lean Cuisine for a home-prepared supper, a bowl of cereal, or two or three eggs over easy to save your stomach the difficulty.

Reconsider Your Dietary Adversaries

How frequently have you struggled through a cup of frozen yogurt while supplicating your stomach doesn't fire misbehaving? Even though you could feel like it's anything but no joking matter to push your body as far as possible, you may be feeling the loss of the foundation of the issue: you could be experiencing a food narrow-mindedness or sensitivity. In this way, each time you eat dairy, gluten, or refined grains, it can add to additional irritation, a debilitated resistant framework, and weight gain. Figure out how to pay attention to everything that your body says to you by keeping note of any uneasiness in a food diary. Or on the other hand attempt a disposal diet — bring in the professionals for help on the off chance that you're encountering one of these signs you ought to see a nutritionist.

Be Boring

You don't need to stay aware of the most recent food patterns and cook your direction through each foodie magazine on the racks to get lean. Attempting to change your routine over and over again can feel monotonous and tedious, which might make you forsake your supper plans and simply request unhealthy takeout. All things being equal, make eating decisions simple by viewing them as a couple of most loved sound, go-to recipes and stick to them so you can get in shape without working out.

Set aside some margin To Chat During Your Meals

Inexpensive food isn't only terrible for you since it's brimming with gross added substances and synthetic compounds; it's additionally because being eaten as fast as possible is unequivocally designed. Furthermore, that is terrible news since you can wind up eating an overabundance to feel full. It requires approximately 20 minutes for your stomach to indicate to your cerebrum that you've eaten your fill. Eat your dinner at superspeed, and you're bound to indulge. Our idea? Set aside some margin to visit with your loved ones while you eat. Put your fork down. Bite gradually. Anything that will broaden your dinner until the 20-minute imprint.

Size Down

It may not be an earth-shattering exhortation, but rather it's time tested: segment control saves you many calories over the long haul. Requesting your number one latte in a tall size rather than a venti can save you something like 150 calories for every Starbucks run. Maintain that more straightforward ways should adhere to serving sizes. Look at these simple methods for controlling piece sizes.

Clear out

Here is one more motivation to skirt the rec center: in addition to the fact that reviews show your body consumes more calories when you practice outside contrasted with inside, however an Environmental Science and Technology investigation as of late observed that you're likewise bound to report a more noteworthy feeling of delight, excitement, and confidence and lower feeling of discouragement, pressure, and exhaustion essentially by strolling in nature contrasted with on a troubling treadmill. Obviously, as a reward you're consuming more calories, however, Cornell specialists have likewise found that working on your psychological well-being and state of mind can prompt better food decisions.

Dole Out Plates Before You Sit

We're tremendous advocates of family suppers, however, make a point to plate your home-prepared dinners before finding a spot at the table. At the point when you feast buffet-style from the counter as opposed to spreading out each dish on the lounge area table, it makes individuals mull over whether they truly need one more aid before getting up to serve themselves once more. At the point when the food is directly before their plate and reachable, it's a lot harder to dismiss it, and family suppers could transform into one of the 50 Little Things Making You increasingly fat.

Eat Eggs In the Morning

Research has shown having eggs for breakfast can cause you to feel all the more full and assist you with eating fewer calories over the day, significance they're an incredible unmistakable advantage for weight reduction. Healthfully talking, one enormous hard-bubbled egg (around 50 grams) contains short of what one gram of carbs and stays a magnificent wellspring of protein. Eggs are additionally stacked with amino acids, cancer prevention agents, and solid fats.

Avoid The Bread Basket

There is no denying supper rolls are scrumptious, however, while feasting out, rather than carb-stacking so from the beginning of the dinner, avoid the bread container and request a verdant green serving of mixed greens all things being equal. On the off chance that the bread container is still too enticing to even consider staying away from, take a stab at crunching on a high-fiber nibble before going out, like a modest bunch of nuts. The fiber found in nuts will keep you satisfied, meaning you will not be as effortlessly actuated to go after the bread and butter, and you'll trade out undesirable fats for solid ones. It's a mutual benefit!

On the off chance that Drinking, Stick To Wine

Similar to drinking your espresso dark, it's essential to keep your beverage orders as straightforward as could be expected. A 2012 CDC investigation discovered that the normal grown-up polishes off around 100 calories worth of liquor day to day, however, inclining toward a glass of wine rather than lager or sweet mixed drinks can decrease that figure and make your waistline slimmer. As well as having fewer calories than most cocktails, red wine, specifically, contains resveratrol, a cell reinforcement that is accepted to have heart medical advantages since it forestalls vein harm and diminishes your 'terrible cholesterol.' Just make sure to soak up with some restraint

Research originally connected TV watching to corpulence quite a while back, and from that point forward extra exploration has been finished to demonstrate how screen time overall (time spent before PCs, iPads, and so forth) can add to weight gain. Since sitting in front of the TV or riding the Internet during dinner can be diverting, a Harvard concentration found it will in general lead individuals to eat more and in this manner consume more calories. All things being equal, specialists exhort turning off during supper time so you can zero in on the thing you are eating, that way you will not gorge and you'll know when you're full.

On the off chance that your clothing regulation permits, wear pants to work. A concentrate by the American Council on Exercise tracked down that easygoing dress, rather than conventional business clothing, can increment actual work levels in one's day-to-day everyday practice. Members in the review made an extra 491 strides and consumed 25 additional calories, on days they sported denim than while wearing conventional work clothing. Even wearing denim on Casual Friday can have an effect. Specialists say keeping it easygoing just once seven days could slice 6,250 calories throughout the year — enough to counterbalance the typical yearly weight gain (0.4 to 1.8 pounds) experienced by most Americans.

Discussing work is no mystery being fastened to a work area all day is terrible for your general wellbeing. Be that as it may, essentially remaining in a work area rather than sitting has been displayed to add to weight reduction. Specialists tracked down standing consumes around 54 calories more than a six-hour day, and albeit that probably won't seem like a lot, those calories collect rapidly. At that rate, you can consume more than

1,000 calories a month by simply remaining on your feet.
In all honesty, a horde of studies has shown that essentially turning down the indoor regulator by a couple of degrees can assist you with getting more fit since cooler temperatures force the body to work harder to remain warm. For a 2013 Japanese review, members were presented to 63 degrees two hours every day for a considerable length of time. At the review's end, their typical muscle-to-fat ratio mass diminished by around five percent.
Regardless of whether have the opportunity and willpower to head out to the exercise center, getting your heart siphoning every day can add to weight reduction. Whether it's taking the canine for a morning walk or utilizing the steps rather than the lift, expanding your pulse even momentarily every day will keep your body solid and in shape, in this manner diminishing undesirable weight gain.

Variety Matters

However it might sound senseless, the shade of your dishware and the shade of your food can decide if you eat pretty much. Per a new report from Cornell University, burger joints serve themselves more food on the off chance that the shade of their food matches the shade of their plate. At the end of the day, on the off chance that you're eating from a white plate, you're bound to take more rice or pasta. On the other hand, assuming you want to eat less, select plates that have high differentiation from what you intend to serve for supper.

Buy Smaller Dishes

Talking about dishes, buying more modest ones can likewise assist you with getting in shape without practice because more modest dishes mean a Moore plaza modest piece size. By topping off a more modest plate, you can fool your cerebrum into believing it's devouring a greater number of calories than it would on the off chance that a similar measure of food was put on a bigger dish.

Have A Larger Breakfast, And Smaller is a teenage girl to get your car Dinner

Presence of mental states to get more fit you shouldn't have an enormous dinner not sometime before hitting the sack, and presently we have an extra examination to back up that speculation. A review distributed in The Obesity Society followed two gatherings of overweight ladies with the metabolic condition on indistinguishable 1,400-calorie weight reduction consumes fewer calories for a considerable length of time. While the two gatherings consumed 500 calories at lunch, one gathering consumed 700 calories for breakfast and a 200-calorie supper (the "enormous breakfast" bunch), while the other gathering had 200 calories at breakfast and 700 calories at supper (the "large supper" bunch). Although the supplement content of the feasts was the very same for the two gatherings, following three months the enormous breakfast bunch lost around twice more weight as the large supper bunch.

Try not to Skip Breakfast

However you might think skirting a dinner, for example, breakfast will assist you with getting more fit since you would be consuming fewer calories, various investigations have shown that abandoning breakfast is terrible for your waistline. "Why," you inquire. It would appear skipping breakfast not just means you'll probably consume more calories later in the day, however eating more calories in the later piece of the day is a bad dream for metabolic circadian rhythms, which assist with holding your weight under tight restraints.

Channel Your Inner Squirrel

On the off chance that you feel yourself getting those early afternoon cravings for food, put down the pop and piece of candy and decide on certain nuts all things being equal. Pecans, almonds, cashews, and Brazil nuts are low in carbs while additionally being magnificent wellsprings of good fats and fiber, meaning they keep you more full longer. As per a concentrate in The Journal of Nutrition, eating almonds with fundamental dinners diminishes a few markers of oxidative harm, which works on your general well-being.

Change From White Potatoes To Sweet Potatoes

Albeit white potatoes offer a few potassium and fiber, yams rule in the nourishment division, so consistently go after yams rather than their white partners. Does an enormous yam contain around 4 grams of satiety-supporting protein, 25% of the day's midsection filling fiber, and multiple times the suggested day-to-day admission of vitamin A. Additionally? It's under 200 calories. On the other hand, a white potato has as many as 250 calories.

Plate Properly

It ought to shock no one that what you put on your plate matters, particularly assuming you're attempting to shed a few pounds. For a reasonable and solid eating regimen, 66% of your supper plate, for instance, ought to comprise lean meats and vegetables — think salmon and broccoli or turkey and spinach. The leftover third can comprise starch, however, and, after it's all said and done hold back nothing like entire grains, lentils, or yams.

Know When To Snack

It's not only essential to nibble strongly over the day, but on the other hand, it's significant to know when you ought to nibble. A review distributed in the Journal of the American Dietetic Association found early in the day snackers ordinarily eat more throughout the day than evening snackers. Besides, specialists found that calorie counters with the early-in-the-day munchies lost a normal of 7% of their absolute body weight while the people who didn't nibble before lunch lost more than 11% of their body weight. That is a distinction of almost 6.5 pounds for a 160-pound lady with a weight reduction objective.

Figure out how To Love Lemon

Not exclusively is drinking lemon water a solid, low-calorie option in contrast to pop or squeeze, however, lemons themselves have likewise been displayed to add to weight reduction. Only one lemon contains a whole day of L-ascorbic acid, a supplement that can diminish levels of cortisol, a pressure chemical that triggers yearning and fat stockpiling. Furthermore, lemons additionally contain polyphenols, which specialists say might avert fat aggregation and weight gain. In all honesty, even the strip is valuable since it is a powerful wellspring of gelatin — a dissolvable fiber that has been demonstrated to assist with peopling feel more full, and longer. As per a review distributed in the Journal of the American College of Nutrition, members who ate only 5 grams of gelatin experienced more satiety.

Embrace Beans

Wheat, Corn, Soybeans, and Oats supermarket

Beans can assist with supporting sensations of completion and overseeing glucose levels, making them a magnificent partner in your weight reduction fight. A new report distributed in The American Journal of Clinical Nutrition found that eating one serving a day of beans, peas, chickpeas or lentils could add to unobtrusive weight reduction. Kidney beans, specifically, are a magnificent wellspring of fiber while likewise being low in carbs, making them an ideal storage space staple for those hoping to shed a couple of pounds.

Drink Cinnamon or Mint Tea

In addition to the fact that tea is a low-calorie option in contrast to espresso-based drinks that will generally be loaded with milk and sugar, however certain assortments of the mitigating refreshment can help add to weight reduction. For instance, Nicole Anziani, MS, RD, CDE, recommends drinking cinnamon tea because the comfortable refreshment might try and assist with diminishing glucose because of cinnamon's impact on blood glucose. Additionally, mint tea can assist with weight reduction since mint is a craving suppressant. A creature concentrated distributed in the Journal of Digestive Diseases found that peppermint oil can loosen up stomach muscles, which can increment the bile stream and work on the assimilation of fats.

Eat Zucchini Noodles Instead Of Pasta

Zucchini noodles seem to be spaghetti, however, the similitudes essentially end there. Eating zoodles over pasta removes void carbs to assist you with getting more fit without working out, however, it additionally adds ever-significant nutrients and fiber. While two cups of pasta contain 480 calories, 90 grams of carbs, and 2 grams of fiber, two cups of zucchini zoodles gloat 66 calories, 12 grams of carbs, and 4 grams of fiber. Whenever arranged well, zoodles can be similarly pretty much as delightful as a bowl of spaghetti, and they can undoubtedly assist you with accomplishing your weight reduction objectives. On the off chance that you want more motivation, take a look at these food trades that cut calories!

PERFECT WEIGHT JOY

With corpulence on the ascent in the United States, (40% are classified as corpulent and 32% are overweight), it's no big surprise Americans have been battling more to get in shape. It's assessed that 45 million individuals in America start an eating routine every year, spending around 33 billion bucks every year. What's more, to exacerbate the situation, a review from the National Weight Control Registry shows that just around 20% of individuals attempting to get in shape figure out how to keep it off over the long haul.

This vertical fight can make it harder for individuals attempting to shed pounds for their well-being and mental self-portrait

issues. In any case, it is essential to comprehend that drawn-out weight reduction is conceivable, and there are unmistakable mental and close-to-home advantages to arriving at that objective. We should get you persuaded with a gander at the positive close-to-home effect a slimmer you can have.
Inhabitants of Beverly Hills, California battling with weight reduction can find support from Dr. Shawn Veiseh, whose training offers far-reaching care for this and different issues with on-location tests, demonstrative tests, and various medicines.
Here are the positive mental and close-to-home effects of weight reduction you can hope to encounter:

Confidence

Such a large amount of our confidence is enveloped by our appearance, which is much of the time supported by certain negative reactions to our weight. Furthermore, on the off chance that you see yourself as ugly, you might expect that is the way everybody sees you, which causes what is happening where you might be less propelled to change since you could see it as purposeless.

Dealing with the confidence issues to arrive at your weight objectives will bring about giving yourself significantly more self-assurance, a more certain self-perception, a superior point of view toward your life, and how others will see you will just build up what you've figured out how to achieve. Individual satisfaction with your self-perception is indispensable to our general prosperity, and this is a major move toward assisting with that.

Personal satisfaction

One of the outcomes of the expansion in overweight and corpulent youngsters and grown-ups is a more serious gamble of a wide range of conditions, like hypertension (hypertension), elevated cholesterol, type 2 diabetes, cardiovascular sickness, stroke, and rest apnea.

The advantages of getting more fit (even just five to 10 %) not just diminish your possibilities of many circumstances, it additionally assists you with dozing better, diminishes pressure, further develops energy, state of mind, imperativeness, and can assist with reestablishing charisma. It can likewise assist with propelling you to be more dynamic and be better ready to do things that will keep you solid.

Pride

This may not seem like a lot, however as we've referenced beforehand, a large number of individuals battle with weight reduction, and under a fourth of them prevail with regards to getting in shape and keeping it off for broadened timeframes. Getting in shape won't just assist you with living better and working on your mental self-portrait, however, it can likewise give a strong feeling of achievement, which can push you to lose more and keep it off.

What's more, to assist you with accomplishing that achievement, we offer a health improvement plan that is planned explicitly to assist you with getting in shape and keeping it off. A blend of wellness assessment, preparation, prescriptions, and dealing with an eating regimen plan are accessible to assist you with arriving at your weight objectives.

Medical advantages

We'll be quick to concede that it's magnificent to slip on a scanty bathing suit and realize you look astonishing in it. In any case, keeping a sound weight (whether that implies dropping a couple of pounds or acquiring some) is about far beyond prompting envy when you're at the pool. Here's the verification.

Diminished Breast Cancer Risk

Being overweight can expand your chances of bosom malignant growth by 30 to 60 percent, as indicated by the Prevent Cancer Foundation. Stomach fat is especially hazardous; it can expand your gamble by 43%

Further developed Heart Health

Research distributed in the Journal of the American College of Cardiology that took a gander at almost 15,000, in any case, sound Korean grown-ups with no known coronary illness found that individuals with a weight record (BMI) of more than 25 were bound to give indications of early plaque development in their supply routes when contrasted with ordinary weight individuals. That's what this made specialists presume, even though these individuals might have been metabolically solid at the hour of the review, their weight was most likely as yet beginning to have unfortunate results on their wellbeing.

distributed in The International Journal of Obesity recommends that overweight ladies' cerebrums answer adversely to working out — however, that the minds of ladies who are at a solid weight are emphatically invigorated by photographs of individuals in a perspiration meeting.

Expanded Fertility

The best weight —, taking everything into account — is a BMI somewhere in the range of 20 and 24, say fruitfulness specialists. The American Society for Reproductive Medicine appraises that 12% of fruitlessness cases are a direct result of weight-related issues (with approximately an equivalent number of individuals experiencing barrenness being overweight and underweight).

Why? Your weight can influence your periods and ovulation — so on the off chance that you're not at solid poundage, your fruitfulness can endure

Better Sleep

As indicated by a recent report from Johns Hopkins University School of Medicine, getting more fit — particularly troublesome stomach fat — can assist you with logging greater Zzs. "Fat, and especially midsection fat, slows down lung capability," says Kerry J. Stewart, Ed.D., a teacher of medication at Johns Hopkins University and one of the review creators. "It becomes more enthusiastically for the lungs to extend because fat is standing out." And since breathing issues can prompt evening time issues like rest apnea, it negatively affects your shuteye.

Diminished Risk of Diabetes

For individuals who are overweight, even minor weight reduction is related to postponing — or forestalling — diabetes, as indicated by the American Diabetes Association.

More Birthday Candles

It's a well-known fact that generally expected weight individuals have a lower chance of infection and in this manner, live longer. Be that as it may, do you know exactly how much longer? The Organization for Economic Co-operation and Development, which has concentrated on the worldwide financial effects of corpulence, expresses that for every 33 pounds of overabundance weight, the gamble of death increments by around 30%. They gauge that the life expectancy of a corpulent individual (that is anybody with a BMI of 40-45) is as long as 10 years more limited than that of an ordinary-weight individual.

www.ingramcontent.com/pod-product-compliance
Lightning Source LLC
LaVergne TN
LVHW052058160826
845678LV00015B/3282